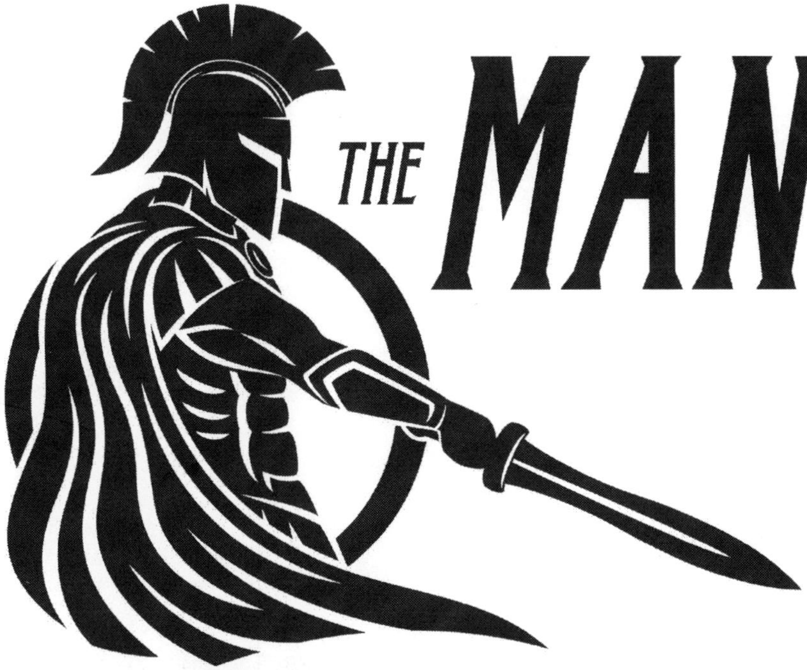

THE MAN

JOURNAL

365 AND ¼ QUESTIONS THAT BUILD COURAGE, CONFIDENCE, AND DISCIPLINE

THE MAN JOURNAL

365 and 1/4 Questions That Build Courage, Confidence, And Discipline

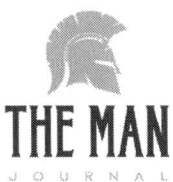

THE MAN
JOURNAL

To all the men who came before us,
and the sacrifices they made.

What's your name, man?

_____

What's your intention with this book? What do you want to get out of it?

_____

_____

_____

_____

One of these questions will change your life forever. Which one will it be?

What will this journal do for you?

This is a journal for men. It includes 365 and ¼ questions that will lead you to self-discovery and unlock your full potential. Writing in this journal means slapping on some war paint and asking tough questions. These questions are designed to spark reflection, growth, and change.

They may also cause you to shed the occasional man tear when no one is looking.

All kidding aside, this book is a hero's journey into the unknown depths of you. It's an exploration of your values and philosophy of life. It will help you express what you truly believe, and draw a map towards a better future. It will help you improve your career, relationships, health, finances, and self-awareness.

The cost of not answering these questions, on the other hand, is painful. It means:

- Staying stuck where you are.

- Failing to grow.

- Missing out on career and financial opportunities.

- Slipping into old patterns of emotions and behavior.

The choice, as always, is yours to make.

How should you use this journal?

I'll suggest three ways, and you can choose your own adventure.

1. Answer one question per day, as prescribed. Take 5-10 minutes and respond in a place where you won't be disturbed. Make it a daily routine. This is the IDEAL option.

2. Take one hour, once a week, and blast through several questions in a sitting. We'll call this the thirsty camel approach. It's not the best option, but hey, that's how life works sometimes.

3. Flip through the book with the greedy eyes of a gold prospector, searching for the good stuff. Mine the gold, and move along. This won't be as helpful, but you'll get *something* out of it.

If these methods aren't ideal for you, then feel free to take complete control and jot down whatever you want.

You're the boss.

Why I wrote this journal

I wrote this journal for myself — because I've struggled with courage, confidence, and discipline in my life. I wanted a set of guiding questions to follow, so that I could reflect on what it means to be a man, and the steps I'd need to take to get there. I quickly found that these questions would be useful to others.

And so this book was born. Its aim is simple: to help guys become men, and men become… well… better men.

The power of questions

There is nothing more powerful in this world than a great question.

Research shows that simply asking people whether they will buy a car, vote for a candidate, or donate blood increases the chances that they will do it. When your brain hears a question, it can't help but think up a response. If it hears the right question, your life can change in wonderful ways.

In my own life, these questions have helped me:

- Wake up early every morning

- Lift heavier weights

- Put together an exit plan to escape my shitty job

- Take charge of my money

- Be more present in my relationships

I have no doubt that the questions you find in this book will help you accomplish goals like these — often things you've been wanting to do for years.

Before you set out on the long, dark journey towards accomplishing your goals, it's good to have a plan. Write down where, when and for how long you intend to write in this book each day/week.

Here is a format I like: *I will (action) at (time) in (location).*

An example: *I will write for 5-10 minutes at 8:30 pm in the office.*

Now it's your turn:

_____

_____

Are you finished? Great.

··●··

It's time to set out on a great adventure. Wealth, happiness, and personal growth lie in wait for you. If you make the effort, you will finish this book a more confident, courageous, and disciplined version of yourself.

What are you waiting for?

"And you? When will you begin that long journey into yourself?"

- **Rumi**

DAY 1

What does being a man mean to you? What qualities or characteristics should a man have?

_____

_____

_____

_____

_____

_____

_____

DAY 2

What would your life look like if you were operating at your full potential, at peak performance?

_____

_____

_____

_____

_____

_____

_____

DAY 3

What is one area of your life that is holding you back, and how could you overcome it?

_____

_____

_____

_____

_____

_____

_____

DAY 4

What two or three things are you most grateful for in life?

_____

_____

_____

_____

_____

_____

_____

DAY 5

If you knew you couldn't fail, what would you set out to do?

_____

_____

_____

_____

_____

_____

DAY 6

If you could have anyone's voice in your head, whose would you choose? What would they say to inspire and motivate you?

_____

_____

_____

_____

_____

DAY 7

What is one of your goals for the next year? If someone put a gun to your head, how would you achieve that goal in the next month?

_____

_____

_____

_____

_____

DAY 8

What would you do if money was no object? How would you spend your days?

_____

_____

_____

_____

_____

_____

DAY 9

What could you do in the next year to make money less of an issue for you? What's your plan? How will you hustle?

_____

_____

_____

_____

_____

DAY 10

What are you thrilled about right now? What makes you so excited about it?

(If you aren't thrilled about anything in particular, what could you be thrilled about if you had to be?)

_____

_____

_____

_____

DAY 11

What difficult conversations are you not having? With whom?

DAY 12

Choose a moment in your life when you felt completely alive. What contributed to that feeling the most?

DAY 13

On a day-to-day basis, are you doing busywork or meaningful work? What can you do to include more meaningful work in your days?

_____

_____

_____

_____

_____

DAY 14

On a scale of 1 to 10, how badly do you want to succeed at your work? How could you get to a 9?

If you're at a 10, what work are you doing each day to make it happen?

_____

_____

_____

_____

DAY 15

What are you afraid of? How has that stopped you before?

How can you prevent it from stopping you in the future?

DAY 16

What are two or three things that put you into a state of flow, where time flies by and you feel fully immersed and involved in what you are doing? Write them down here.

DAY 17

How important is self-improvement to you? What are the costs of not changing?

_____

_____

_____

_____

_____

_____

_____

DAY 18

Are you a hero or a victim in your own story?

What can you do to get out of the victim mindset and move towards the hero mindset?

_____

_____

_____

_____

_____

_____

DAY 19

When you are 90 years old and lying on your deathbed, what do you think your biggest regrets will be?

_____

_____

_____

_____

_____

_____

_____

DAY 20

What can you do tomorrow that will make you feel proud at the end of the day? Make a plan, and take action.

_____

_____

_____

_____

_____

DAY 21

What major decisions do you have coming up? What resources (time, feedback, energy, etc.) do you need to make an optimal decision?

DAY 22

What makes you forget to eat or go to the bathroom? How can you do it in a way that helps other people?

DAY 23

How do you wish the world was different? If you could change anything about it, what would you change?

DAY 24

Make a list of all the 'superpowers' you have. Dig deep.

DAY 25

What do you think matters more: happiness or meaning? Why is that?

_____

_____

_____

_____

_____

_____

DAY 26

When are you most "yourself"? What are you doing when you feel like that?

_____

_____

_____

_____

_____

_____

DAY 27

What have you been put on this earth to create? If you're not sure, have a quick brainstorm.

DAY 28

Have you ever pushed yourself to your limits in your work or play? Do you know where your limits are in a day?

Most people never discover what they are truly capable of. What can you do to make sure that won't be you?

DAY 29

How much potential do you have, in the different areas of your abilities? In what ways could you realize that potential?

DAY 30

What are you most curious about? How can you follow your curiosity more?

"Waste no more time arguing what a good man should be. Be one."

- Marcus Aurelius

DAY 31

What are you most proud of? Make a list of things you've accomplished that fill you with strength and self-esteem.

DAY 32

Who are your personal heroes? What have they done to inspire you?

DAY 33

Tim Ferriss writes that "reality is largely negotiable." How can you negotiate with reality more creatively in order to live a better life?

_____

_____

_____

_____

_____

_____

DAY 34

What can you forgive other people for, that is holding you back in your life? What can you forgive yourself for that is holding you back?

_____

_____

_____

_____

_____

DAY 35

Write down all the ways that you are self-reliant.

DAY 36

What opportunities are you saying "no" to in life? Why?

(It's okay to say "no" if you are focused on things that matter more.)

DAY 37

Take a few minutes to notice where your body and mind are in space and time. When you are ready, consider this question:

What state are you in right now? ("Ohio" is not a valid answer)

DAY 38

What are two or three goals you want to achieve in the next three years?

DAY 39

What can you do with your time that is important to you and others? What is stopping you from doing it now?

DAY 40

What struggles are you willing to tolerate to get what you want?

DAY 41

If you were selling your own product or service, what would it be? If you already have a product or service, what else could you offer?

_____

_____

_____

_____

_____

DAY 42

How can you show up for the next 48 hours as your best self?

_____

_____

_____

_____

_____

_____

DAY 43

What questions do you need to start asking yourself each day in order to live a better life?

_____

_____

_____

_____

_____

_____

_____

DAY 44

What does your ideal morning routine look like? How could you take one small step towards it, starting tomorrow?

_____

_____

_____

_____

_____

DAY 45

Are you good at setting boundaries with people in your life? How could you get better at it?

DAY 46

Write down three self-limiting beliefs that interfere with your life. Now cross them out and replace them with empowering beliefs.

DAY 47

What role do mistakes and failures play in your life? How can you put them to better use?

_____

_____

_____

_____

_____

_____

_____

DAY 48

What does love mean to you? What does it mean to truly love someone?

_____

_____

_____

_____

_____

_____

_____

DAY 49

When you were a child, what were you obsessed with?
How can you channel that obsession now?

DAY 50

Imagine you are in a crowded room at a party. What
do you know that others don't? How could you share
that knowledge?

DAY 51

What kind of legacy do you want to leave behind?
How do you want to be remembered?

DAY 52

What is your idea of personal hell? What suffering do
you want to avoid at all costs?

DAY 53

What is your idea of paradise? What ideal future do you want to move towards?

DAY 54

What problems are you avoiding in your life? How can you address them head on?

DAY 55

Think through a problem in your life from the perspective of one of your personal heroes. What advice would they give you?

_____

_____

_____

_____

_____

_____

DAY 56

If you had your own TV show, what would it be about?

_____

_____

_____

_____

_____

_____

DAY 57

If you wrote a book, what would it be about?

DAY 58

Think of one or two times when you were stronger than you thought you were. What was your reaction? How could you be stronger in other situations?

DAY 59

Imagine a miracle takes place while you are sleeping tonight, and your problems are solved. How will you know the miracle happened when you wake up?

DAY 60

How would a friend, co-worker, or relative describe you if they were being generous? How about if they were being critical?

"Masculinity is not something given to you, it's something you gain. And you gain it by winning small battles with honor."

-Norman Mailer

DAY 61

On a scale of 1 to 10, how much self-discipline do you have? How could you bring that number closer to 10?

DAY 62

If time is your most valuable resource, what can you do to better protect it? What are you doing now to waste it?

DAY 63

What one new skill would improve your life the most? How would it change things?

DAY 64

What is something that seems to come naturally to you? Describe it in detail.

DAY 65

Set a timer for 5 minutes. Make a list of all the things in your life that you are grateful for.

DAY 66

Write a short letter to your 10-year-old self. What advice would you give him?

DAY 67

If you had a time machine for a day, what year, or period of history, would you travel to? Why?

_____

_____

_____

_____

_____

_____

DAY 68

Set a timer for 5 minutes. Brainstorm on ways you could improve your relationships with family and friends.

_____

_____

_____

_____

_____

DAY 69

What is the biggest change you need to make in order to achieve your goals?

_____

_____

_____

_____

_____

_____

_____

DAY 70

What lessons can you learn from your greatest failures?

_____

_____

_____

_____

_____

_____

_____

DAY 71

What can you get 1% better at today? Could you do it in 5 minutes or less?

DAY 72

Will the habits you have right now lead you to the future you desire? What new habits do you need to develop?

DAY 73

What are your core values? Pick two or three of them and ask: "how can I act on these values?

DAY 74

Which area of your life could benefit from more delayed gratification?

DAY 75

Do you have a bias toward thinking or toward action? How can you reset your default so you take action more?

DAY 76

What do you want more: to improve the world or to enjoy the world? What is your ideal balance between the two?

DAY 77

Which is more important to you: imagination or intelligence? Why?

_____

_____

_____

_____

_____

_____

_____

DAY 78

In what areas of your life are you waiting on the sidelines? How can you jump in and start taking action?

_____

_____

_____

_____

_____

_____

_____

DAY 79

Imagine you were alone in a cabin in the woods for a year. How would you fill your time? What activities or projects would you find to keep busy?

_____

_____

_____

_____

_____

_____

DAY 80

What would happen if you approached your hobby or sport like a full-time job? What could you accomplish?

_____

_____

_____

_____

_____

_____

DAY 81

If you could send a written message to everyone in the world, what would you say? The catch: it has to be 50 words or less.

_____

_____

_____

_____

_____

DAY 82

What is a lesson your parents taught you, that you are grateful for?

_____

_____

_____

_____

_____

_____

_____

DAY 83

What are the main ingredients of a well-lived life to you? What does it mean to live well?

DAY 84

How can you be more present and mindful during the day? What are some techniques you can use?

DAY 85

Whose expectations are you trying to live up to? What are they? How do you feel about them?

_____

_____

_____

_____

_____

_____

DAY 86

What is your strongest "why" in life?

_____

_____

_____

_____

_____

_____

DAY 87

If you could choose any five people to surround yourself with, who would they be?

DAY 88

Who challenges you the most in your life? How do they do it?

DAY 89

What percentage of the average day do you spend in your comfort zone? How much time do you spend each day pushing yourself out of it?

DAY 90

What plans would you make if you knew you would live for another 1,000 years?

"How long are you going to wait before you demand the best of yourself?"

– Epicurus

DAY 91

Three years from now, what will you wish you had done today?

DAY 92

Have you ever had a traumatic experience or a breakdown? How did you grow from it?

DAY 93

What have you learned from the past few years with COVID? (About yourself, your relationships, the world, etc.)

_____

_____

_____

_____

_____

_____

DAY 94

Describe your dark side. What ways can you use to tame it and control it? How can you channel it toward something useful?

_____

_____

_____

_____

_____

_____

DAY 95

What would it take for you to be thrilled about life? If you're already thrilled, what can you do to share this with others?

DAY 96

What is your default way of looking at situations in life? Optimistic, pessimistic? Realistic, artistic? What adjustments could you make in the way you look at things?

DAY 97

What beliefs have you had about the world that were wrong? How often do you update your view of the world?

DAY 98

What is money to you? What is your relationship with money?

DAY 99

Take a problem in your life and imagine it was
happening to someone else. What advice would you
give them?

_____

_____

_____

_____

_____

DAY 100

What is something you are often angry about? Are
there ways you can change it?

_____

_____

_____

_____

_____

DAY 101

How would you describe yourself in five minutes or less? What kind of person are you?

DAY 102

What important lessons do you think the world is trying to teach you?

DAY 103

Are you a human being having a spiritual experience, or a spiritual being having a human experience? What the hell might that even mean?

DAY 104

What is your philosophy of life in five minutes or less? What is most important?

DAY 105

What do you think is the biggest threat to humanity?

How can you prevent it single-handedly? (Just kidding…kind of.)

DAY 106

How long would you survive a zombie apocalypse? What would your strategy be?

DAY 107

How optimistic are you about the future? Why?

DAY 108

When was the last time you laughed so hard that you cried? Try to remember that moment in detail. What sparked it?

DAY 109

Write down this question on a slip of paper: "Am I going to persist in the face of adversity today?" Read it when you wake up tomorrow morning, and again several times during the day.

What impact do you think this will have?

DAY 110

If you had one year left to live, where would you go? How would you spend your time?

DAY 111

We have more than 60,000 thoughts in a day. 90% of those thoughts are repeated from the day before.

What repetitive thoughts do you have? What new thoughts do you think would serve you best?

DAY 112

If you were an architect, what kind of building would you design? Who would it be for? Why?

DAY 113

How likely are you to get enough exercise this week?
How can you make it more likely?

DAY 114

What would an ultra-successful person do if they were
in your shoes? Jot down a few actions they would take.

DAY 115

When was the last time you felt truly heard? How can you give other people that wonderful experience?

DAY 116

What could you invest $100 or $500 in to improve your quality of life right now?

DAY 117

If you wanted to change the way you think about your problems, where would you start?

DAY 118

What questions have you stopped asking the people you love? Why?

DAY 119

Do you run the day, or does the day run you? How can you take charge of today as well as tomorrow?

DAY 120

If you had a full-time life coach, what would they tell you? What would they ask you to do?

"The quality of your life is a direct reflection of the quality of the questions you are asking yourself."

- Tony Robbins

DAY 121

What are you doing when you use your imagination the most? How could you use it more?

DAY 122

Are you the same person you were a year ago? What's changed? What kind of person will you be in a year from now?

DAY 123

How heavy do you think an adult male silverback gorilla is? Guess first, and then see how close you were.

DAY 124

If you could sit down and have dinner with any historical figure, who would you choose? Why?

DAY 125

How might your suffering be the product of your imagination or habitual thinking, and not external reality?

_____

_____

_____

_____

_____

DAY 126

If having a productive day meant getting only one thing done, what would that be? How can you make sure you do that thing each day?

_____

_____

_____

_____

_____

DAY 127

What are you an expert on? What could you become an expert on in five years?

DAY 128

What advice do you think a Buddhist monk would give you? How could you follow it?

DAY 129

Imagine that tomorrow will repeat on a loop, like the movie *Groundhog Day*. What would you want to do on a day that you'd be okay with repeating forever?

DAY 130

Write down some doubts or negative thoughts you've been having recently.

For each one, ask yourself: "Is it true? Or just an opinion?"

Bonus: write "Is it true?" on a paper, and carry it around with you. Every time you catch yourself worrying, pull out the paper and read the question.

DAY 131

Santiago Ramón y Caja wrote *"Any man could, if he were so inclined, be the sculptor of his own brain."*

What kind of brain do you want to have? How can you program it with the right thoughts, intentions, and feelings?

DAY 132

How can you aim for the highest possible good? For yourself, your family and friends, other people in general, and the world, as you prioritize them.

DAY 133

If you had a superhuman level of focus, what would you concentrate on?

DAY 134

What should you put on your "avoid-at-all-costs" list?

DAY 135

What story are you telling yourself about your life? You are holding the pen—you can change the story.

DAY 136

Write a letter to someone in your life who spends a lot of time alone. How can you bring them joy and happiness with your words?

DAY 137

What is easy to concentrate on and gives you energy? What is hard to concentrate on and makes you unfocused?

How can you fill your life with more of the first, and less of the second?

DAY 138

If you could, how would you turn your biggest fears or avoidances into your biggest assets?

DAY 139

Imagine your ideal work environment. What does it look like? Who is in it? What are you doing?

DAY 140

Describe a time in your life where you felt fearlessly creative. What was that like?

DAY 141

If you could ask one of your heroes a single question, what would it be? Write down three questions, and pick the best one.

_____

_____

_____

_____

_____

_____

DAY 142

Are you on the path towards financial freedom, or do you spend more than you make each month? How can you get on track, or move closer to your financial goals?

_____

_____

_____

_____

_____

_____

DAY 143

Which of your strengths are you most proud of? How does it show up in everyday life?

DAY 144

What question could you ask yourself every morning to live an extraordinary life?

DAY 145

Think of an important project or career goal. Imagine that, one year from now, it has failed. What went wrong? What derailed you?

_____

_____

_____

_____

_____

DAY 146

What was your experience with formal education? What would you change about the education system if you could?

_____

_____

_____

_____

_____

DAY 147

Who inspires you to do—and be—better in your life?
Why?

_____

_____

_____

_____

_____

_____

DAY 148

What is your sleep hygiene like? How could you
improve the quality of your sleep?

_____

_____

_____

_____

_____

_____

DAY 149

Do you have strong male friendships? How might you develop healthy bonds with more like-minded men?

_____

_____

_____

_____

_____

_____

DAY 150

How can you better control your social media use, so it doesn't control you?

_____

_____

_____

_____

_____

_____

"Knowing yourself is the beginning of all wisdom."

— **Aristotle**

DAY 151

Henry Ford once said "Whether you think you can or think you can't, you're right."

What do you think you can do, if you put your mind to it?

_____

_____

_____

_____

_____

DAY 152

What is something you are doing well? What is contributing to your success at it?

_____

_____

_____

_____

_____

_____

DAY 153

What do you believe you need in life in order to be truly happy?

DAY 154

What is your worldview? How do you see yourself in the bigger picture?

DAY 155

How are you unique? What peculiar mix of experiences and traits do you have?

DAY 156

Who do you need to lead, in your life? (This can be in small ways like encouraging others.) What could you do to become a better leader?

DAY 157

First, write about one of your biggest insecurities.

Done?

Okay, now challenge the shit out of it.

_____

_____

_____

_____

_____

_____

DAY 158

What might be the root cause of your relationship problems? Your money problems? Now's the time to do some digging.

_____

_____

_____

_____

_____

_____

DAY 159

What are you putting off until tomorrow? Is there a way you can do it today?

DAY 160

Who do you hate with the fire of a thousand suns? Now ask: What lessons can you learn from this person?

DAY 161

When was the last time you had a powerful conversation? What was it about? Who was it with?

DAY 162

What can you do to truly rest and recover at the end of each day? What rituals could you start or maintain?

DAY 163

How can you step outside the cage of your parents' judgment and expectations?

_____

_____

_____

_____

_____

_____

DAY 164

How do you think a woman should be treated? What rules or guidelines can you think of?

_____

_____

_____

_____

_____

_____

DAY 165

What could you create if you gave yourself permission to be bad at it?

DAY 166

What rules do you hold yourself to? What rules do you think you should hold yourself to?

DAY 167

Do you believe you are a fast learner or a slow learner? How might that belief influence you?

_____

_____

_____

_____

_____

_____

DAY 168

Who is your mentor? What have you learned from him or her? If you don't have a mentor, how might you find one?

_____

_____

_____

_____

_____

_____

DAY 169

Take a quick look around you. Every object and technology you see was thought of and created by someone who was often no smarter than you.

What implications does this fact have for you?

DAY 170

What role does perfectionism play in your life? How could you change what you believe about the need for perfection so you can get more done in less time, even if it isn't "perfect"?

DAY 171

What would it mean for you to have a healthy, strong body? Describe what you would look like, and how you would feel.

_____

_____

_____

_____

_____

DAY 172

What are you most looking forward to in your future life? Visualize it as if it were happening right now. How do you feel?

_____

_____

_____

_____

_____

DAY 173

If you could change one thing about the way you were brought up, what would you change?

DAY 174

Imagine that you are 80 years old and telling your life story to your grandchildren. What part of the story are you living now? What will the triumphant part be?

DAY 175

What's in your control in life? What's outside of your control? What should you focus on?

DAY 176

What role does physical excellence (exercise, physical skills, nutrition) have in being a man? How can you improve your life in these areas?

DAY 177

What life event has most significantly shaped who you are as a person? Why?

DAY 178

What weakness do you have that is getting in the way of your progress? How can you confront it?

DAY 179

What does it mean to be a high-value man? Are you one? How could you become one?

DAY 180

Are you okay working for other people? Or would you rather make the sacrifices to work for yourself? Why?

"Every action you take is a vote for the type of person you'd like to become."

- James Clear

DAY 181

If you were an inventor, what invention would you come up with? What would it do?

DAY 182

When was the last time someone asked you a thought-provoking question? What did they ask you?

DAY 183

How might your subconscious mind be sabotaging you? How can you make sure that your mind helps and supports you?

DAY 184

What question should you ask yourself every night before sleeping?

Write that question down and put it beside your bed.

DAY 185

On a scale of 1 to 10, how well do you manage stress?
What would take you closer to a 10?

DAY 186

Visualize yourself reaching one of your biggest goals.
Describe what you see, hear, feel, etc.

DAY 187

What do you think the purpose of meditation is?
What could/does it do for you?

DAY 188

If you had complete self-control, what would your diet
be? What foods would you eat? What foods would you
avoid?

DAY 189

How do you think your thoughts shape your reality?

_____
_____
_____
_____
_____
_____
_____
_____

DAY 190

What do you enjoy doing that other people consider work? What do you enjoy about it?

_____
_____
_____
_____
_____
_____
_____

DAY 191

What is something you can do to increase your sense of connection with other people?

DAY 192

What type of person do you want to be? Which actions bring you closer to being that ideal person? Which actions take you farther away from it?

DAY 193

If you felt like it, what evidence could you find that you are:

- kind?
- generous?
- strong?

DAY 194

What does courage mean to you? When have you been courageous?

DAY 195

Who do you love in life? What are you doing about it?

DAY 196

How can you celebrate the good things in your life more often?

DAY 197

What is the best piece of advice you have ever received? Why did it resonate with you?

DAY 198

What is something about you that would surprise most people? Why would they be surprised?

DAY 199

What is one character trait that you think holds you back in life? How can you change it?

DAY 200

If you were a life coach, what would you ask your clients to help them change their behavior? Try to think of two or three questions.

DAY 201

Which compliment do you most like to receive? What do you think this says about you?

_____

_____

_____

_____

_____

_____

_____

DAY 202

In what areas of life do you give up too easily? In what areas do you persist, even when things get tough? Are there any areas where you persist beyond what is reasonable?

_____

_____

_____

_____

DAY 203

What act of courage have you witnessed? What made it courageous?

DAY 204

What is a lesson in life that you had to learn the hard way? How can you help others avoid this pain?

DAY 205

If you could only ask one question to get to know someone, what question would you ask?

_____

_____

_____

_____

_____

_____

DAY 206

Here are two questions from Anthony Metivier that cut through the bullshit of overthinking:

- Is this thought useful?
- How do thoughts behave?

When do you think you should ask yourself these two questions?

_____

_____

_____

DAY 207

What is something that you would benefit from saying "no" to more?

DAY 208

Do you take enough risks, or do you avoid them? Would you benefit from risking more or less in life?

DAY 209

What do you think is the role of arguments in relationships? How should people disagree?

DAY 210

If you had to leave the house for 10 hours every day, where would you go? What would you do?

"Every strike brings me closer to the next home run."

- Babe Ruth

DAY 211

How much control do you think you have over your destiny? How could you gain more control?

_____

_____

_____

_____

_____

_____

DAY 212

Three core questions in life are:

1. Where do you want to be?

2. What do you want to do?

3. Who do you want to do it with?

Considering where you are right now in life, how do you answer these?

_____

_____

DAY 213

What do you think the role of play is in your life?
Why is it important to play? Are you doing it enough,
not enough, or too much?

DAY 214

What do you think the world will be like in 50 years?
What can you do to prepare for it?

What can you do to help create it?

DAY 215

If you were called in to teach a 10th grade class, what would you teach them? What lesson or question would you want to leave them with?

DAY 216

Would you prefer $1,000 today, or $10,000 in 10 years? Why?

DAY 217

If you went to college: What class do you wish you had taken but didn't? What interests you about it?

If you're in college now, you're in luck! Go take that course.

DAY 218

What do you think is the biggest obstacle to your happiness? What are some ways you could work on overcoming that obstacle?

DAY 219

What is your inner compass? What direction does it point to?

DAY 220

What do you wish someone would remind you about daily?

DAY 221

How would your life be different if you didn't own a smartphone? Or a computer?

If you don't have one or both of those, what would happen if you did?

_____

_____

_____

_____

_____

DAY 222

Set a timer for 5 minutes. Without stopping, write about your ideal self.

Read what you just wrote. What surprises you?

_____

_____

_____

_____

_____

DAY 223

In what ways are you weird? How can you use your
weirdness in a way that benefits your life?

DAY 224

What technology doesn't exist in the world, but
should?

DAY 225

What 20% of effort in your life is bringing you 80% of the results? How can you focus on that 20% more effectively?

_____

_____

_____

_____

_____

DAY 226

Do you wake up as soon as your alarm goes off, or do you snooze?

What would make you more thrilled to get up in the morning?

_____

_____

_____

_____

DAY 227

If you were suddenly the CEO of a company, which company would you choose? What would be the first change you'd make?

DAY 228

Who—or what—is backing you into a corner? How can you become a credible adversary to it and take action?

DAY 229

How would you act today if you believed in yourself unconditionally?

DAY 230

What are you most afraid of missing out on in life? What actions can you take to make sure you don't miss out?

DAY 231

What is something you believe that most people would disagree with? What reasons do you have for believing it?

_____

_____

_____

_____

_____

DAY 232

How decisive are you? What can you do to get more practice at this crucial skill?

_____

_____

_____

_____

_____

DAY 233

Which animal do you admire the most? What traits does it have?

_____
_____
_____
_____
_____
_____
_____

DAY 234

Consider a current problem in your life. Ask yourself: what would Batman do in this situation? (Or another superhero, if Batman doesn't inspire you.)

_____
_____
_____
_____
_____
_____

DAY 235

What three areas do you spend most of your money on? Are there any leaks in your financial ship? What are they?

DAY 236

Which two supplements could you take every day to improve your brain and heart health? When would you take them?

DAY 237

What mountains in life do you most want to climb? Are you climbing the right mountain right now?

DAY 238

What would it take for you to break into the top 1% of your field? How about the top 1% of your hobby or sport?

DAY 239

What are the downsides to using pornography? Make a list.

How can you strengthen your self-discipline—instead of your forearm?

_____

_____

_____

_____

_____

DAY 240

What, or who, is your biggest source of inspiration?

_____

_____

_____

_____

_____

_____

"If there is no struggle, there is no progress."

- Frederick Douglass

DAY 241

What is one of your most prized possessions? Why is it important to you?

_____

_____

_____

_____

_____

_____

DAY 242

If you had to move to a different country tonight, which one would you choose? What draws you to that country?

_____

_____

_____

_____

_____

DAY 243

What are you keeping track of and measuring in your life? As Peter Drucker said: "Only what gets measured, gets managed."

DAY 244

What are you doing for others? Martin Luther King called this "life's most persistent and urgent question."

DAY 245

What thoughts keep you up at night? How can you best deal with them during the day, so you can get a good night's sleep?

_____

_____

_____

_____

_____

_____

DAY 246

In what ways are you a devil?

_____

_____

_____

_____

_____

_____

_____

DAY 247

Life is going to throw lots of adversity and struggles your way. How can you prepare for them?

DAY 248

What am are you missing by choosing to worry or be afraid? (source: Ryan Holiday)

DAY 249

In what areas of life are you competing with other people? What are they doing that you're not doing?

DAY 250

How do you deal with bullies and assholes in life? What are effective strategies?

DAY 251

On a scale of 1 to 10, how good are your time management skills? What would it take to get them closer to a 10?

DAY 252

If you could be part of something greater than yourself (or what you're currently doing), what would it be? What organization would you join?

DAY 253

What kind of self-care routines do you have?
Meditation, yoga, exercise?

What takes you from "wired" to relaxed in 10
minutes?

DAY 254

What sacrifices would it take to live the life of your
dreams?

DAY 255

What is your relationship to things like alcohol, drugs, food, sugar, and caffeine? What is a healthier approach you could take in this area of life?

DAY 256

How can you make sure your money is working for you, so at some point you won't have to work for money? What is your investment strategy?

DAY 257

If you had to treat yourself like someone you were responsible for helping, how would you act differently? (source: Jordan Peterson)

DAY 258

What do you think drives people to do evil things? How can you avoid doing evil things yourself?

DAY 259

If you were the last person on earth, how would you find meaning and fulfillment? Would it be possible?

DAY 260

Imagine that you are attending a ceremony where you are receiving a major award. What would you like it to be for?

DAY 261

What would happen if you only said things that were completely true?

DAY 262

What book, movie, or documentary would you recommend to someone who is suffering? What lessons do you think it can teach?

DAY 263

What is the next chapter of your life story? Write it down in 30-50 words.

DAY 264

Describe the most incredible day of your entire life. What happened? What made it so great?

DAY 265

On a scale of 1 to 10, how much do you procrastinate? What actions can you take to get that number closer to 1?

DAY 266

What role does anxiety play in your life? How can you reframe your anxiety?

DAY 267

What are you most hopeful about in life?

DAY 268

If you had to go up on a stage and do 5 minutes of stand-up comedy, what would you talk about to get laughs?

DAY 269

If you were a philosopher looking for the meaning of life, what unexpected place might you look?

DAY 270

Think about a highly successful person in your field. If they can do it, why not you? What would happen if you did what they did for one year?

"We must all suffer from one of two pains: the pain of discipline or the pain of regret. The difference is discipline weighs ounces while regret weighs tons."

- Jim Rohn

DAY 271

Make a list of things that scare you. Choose a small fear, and go out and face it. Then, face another one… then another one… and keep going until you've faced a major one.

DAY 272

What habit in your life are you most proud of? What habit do you want to lose?

DAY 273

What do you think women are looking for in a man? How can you embody those qualities more?

DAY 274

What is something that most people accept as true or self-evident that you think is total BS?

DAY 275

What do you plan to do with your one wild and precious life? (source: Mary Oliver)

DAY 276

How much does it matter to you what other people think of you? How does that affect your choices and behaviors in life?

DAY 277

Have you ever gone broke or been extremely poor?
What steps can you take to avoid poverty?

DAY 278

What would you do if you needed to increase your
results by 10X next year? What steps would you take?

DAY 279

How often do you compare yourself to others? How often do you compare yourself to past versions of you?

DAY 280

When was the last time you cried man tears? What were the reasons and what was the situation?

DAY 281

Which is more important to you: wisdom or money?
Why?

DAY 282

What are you holding onto that you might want to let
go of? What fucks do you want to stop giving?

DAY 283

What does it mean to be human? What excites you most about being human?

_____

_____

_____

_____

_____

_____

DAY 284

If you aren't doing what you love yet, how might you love what you're doing? How could you love your job more?

_____

_____

_____

_____

_____

DAY 285

What small act of kindness has someone done for you that had a big impact?

DAY 286

Do you live your life inwardly or outwardly? How can you strike a balance between the two?

DAY 287

What five words would you use to describe your future self in five years?

_____

_____

_____

_____

_____

_____

DAY 288

If you had 10 minutes left to live, what message would you want to leave for the people you love? Write it down here (and keep a box of man tissues nearby).

_____

_____

_____

_____

_____

DAY 289

If you could know the answer to any question in the world, what would it be? Why?

DAY 290

If you had to sleep 16 hours a night and only had 8-hour days, how would you prioritize your time?

DAY 291

If your life depended on it, could you accomplish something important for the human race in the next two years? What would you do?

_____

_____

_____

_____

_____

DAY 292

Who is someone you should say "no" to more often? Plan how you can do this.

What are the different ways you can say "no"? (One of my go-to phrases is _"That doesn't work for me."_)

_____

_____

_____

_____

DAY 293

What place in the world has impacted you the most? Visualize it in your mind's eye. How did it change you?

DAY 294

If you had a crystal ball and could see one hundred years into the future, what would you be most curious about? Where would you look?

DAY 295

Do you think being overconfident is useful? What are the pros and cons of being overconfident?

DAY 296

How worthy do you feel of love and kindness? How about success and wealth? What would make you feel more worthy?

DAY 297

Do you approach the world from a place of scarcity or abundance? What beliefs contribute to that mindset?

DAY 298

How much money would make you financially free? Do you have a number in mind? If not, that's okay— do a quick brainstorm and figure it out.

DAY 299

How much is your time worth? What would you like your aspirational hourly rate to be?

DAY 300

Are we living in a giant simulation? Yes or yes? All kidding aside, what would it mean if we were?

"Being male is a matter of birth. Being a man is a matter of choice."

-Edwin Louis Cole

DAY 301

What do you like to do when no one is around? What can you learn about yourself from that?

DAY 302

What makes someone a genius? Is it something you are born with, or can you develop it?

DAY 303

Which challenge, or challenges, in your life are you most grateful for? Why?

DAY 304

Where do you have your best ideas? How can you have more of them?

DAY 305

What is something new that you could try today?
Bonus high-five if you get up and go do it!

DAY 306

Do you have a growth mindset, or a fixed mindset?
What's the difference?

DAY 307

What are the biggest distractions in your life? Come up with an action plan to manage them.

DAY 308

Have you ever burned out from too much work or stress? How did you recover? How can you prevent future burnouts?

DAY 309

Some of your firmly held beliefs about the world are false. Which ones might they be? How might you find out?

DAY 310

What do you know for sure to be true? How do you know it?

DAY 311

Consider an important goal that you have. Under what conditions would it be okay to give up on it? Why?

DAY 312

Make a list of the things a "hero" might do in a day. Then, make a list of all the things a "loser" does.

How can you have more "hero" days?

DAY 313

What will your future self thank you for in five years?
What will he be angry at you for?

DAY 314

What one skill could you learn that would pay the
biggest dividends? What actions can you take today to
start learning it?

DAY 315

How much sex is ideal for you? How often would you like to have a "roll in the hay"?

DAY 316

What is your biggest health concern? What steps can you take to manage it?

DAY 317

If you had to write one sentence that captures your mission in life, what would you write?

DAY 318

Consider a difficult problem or upcoming decision in your life. Ask yourself:

1. What does my head say?

2. What does my heart say?

3. What does my gut say?

DAY 319

How much time alone do you need? Are you getting enough? More than you want?

DAY 320

If you are stuck in a job/relationship/life situation that you aren't happy with, what's your escape plan?

DAY 321

What is something you can offer the world that no one else can offer?

DAY 322

How do you deal with unexpected events? How can you improve the way you deal with them?

DAY 323

On a scale of 1 to 10, how good are you at problem-solving? What would bring you closer to a 10?

DAY 324

What triggers your anger the most? What can you do to not get caught off-guard?

DAY 325

The psychiatrist Viktor Frankl identified three sources of meaning in life: your work, your relationships, and the way you face suffering.

Which source of meaning is most important to you? How can you develop in these three areas?

_____

_____

_____

_____

DAY 326

Do you think we discover ourselves or create ourselves? What steps can you take toward self-discovery or self-creation?

_____

_____

_____

_____

_____

DAY 327

What pain do you face on a daily basis?

Can you change it? Can you change the way you see it, or feel about it?

DAY 328

Think of a problem you are facing. How would a ninja tackle it? How would a military general tackle it?

DAY 329

If you had an alter ego, who would it be? Why?

DAY 330

If you could instantly develop three qualities, what would they be? (Some examples: being hardworking, persistent, tidy, decisive.) Why?

"*I mean to make myself a man, and if I succeed in that, I shall succeed in everything else.*"

- James A. Garfield

DAY 331

Cal Newport says "focus is the new IQ."

What step can you take right now to develop greater focus?

_____

_____

_____

_____

_____

DAY 332

Important question:

Why is it that we call bacon "bacon," and cookies "cookies," when we cook bacon and bake cookies?

_____

_____

_____

_____

_____

DAY 333

Ray Dalio writes that "pain + reflection = progress."
What pain can you reflect on right now to make
progress?

_____

_____

_____

_____

_____

DAY 334

How does your inner warrior look? talk? act?

How can you tap into that inner warrior state more
often?

_____

_____

_____

_____

_____

DAY 335

Do you keep score in life based on what others want, or what you want? What can you do to develop an inner "scorecard?"

DAY 336

In what areas of your life are you avoiding feedback? How can you seek it out more often so you can get better?

DAY 337

How would you describe your self-image? How flexible might your concept of "self" be?

DAY 338

What would you be happy to do for 14 hours a day, 7 days a week?

DAY 339

What fears have you overcome in your life? How were you able to do it?

_____

_____

_____

_____

_____

_____

DAY 340

How comfortable are you with uncertainty? What steps can you take to embrace or accept it more?

_____

_____

_____

_____

_____

_____

DAY 341

What effort or actions fill you with confidence? How can you make them a regular part of your day?

DAY 342

When have you felt "whole"? What contributed to that feeling? Describe the experience.

DAY 343

What does your inner critic often say? How can you effectively tell it to fuck off?

DAY 344

What is something you feel ashamed about? How can you let go of that shame?

DAY 345

Imagine there is an apple in your hand. Visualize it. What does it look like? What color, shape, texture? Try to smell it.

Now, take a bite of the imaginary apple.

What did you experience?

If your mind can make that seem real, what else can it do?

DAY 346

Who are you being right now, and is that the person you want to be? What might you change?

DAY 347

In what areas of your life are you drifting right now? How can you take charge?

DAY 348

Do you think you can become funnier? How would you do that?

DAY 349

How can you approach life more like a gift?

DAY 350

If you wrote a checklist for your perfect day, what would be on it?

DAY 351

What dreams have you given up on? What happened to make you give up?

DAY 352

How comfortable are you with being uncomfortable? How could you embrace discomfort more?

DAY 353

What sacrifices did your ancestors make for you? How can you honor them for what they have given you?

DAY 354

If you died and then came back as a new person, animal, plant, or thing, who or what would it be? Why?

DAY 355

If everything you wrote about your future came true, what would you write? Take a few minutes and write down your ideal future in broad strokes.

_____

_____

_____

_____

_____

DAY 356

What things can you do better than your past self today? Have a quick brainstorm.

_____

_____

_____

_____

_____

DAY 357

What ideas do you love? How can you make them part of your daily routine, like showering, or brushing your teeth, or shitting?

DAY 358

What are your thoughts on work-life balance? Is there anything worth unbalancing your life for?

DAY 359

What secrets do you feel like you know about how the world works?

DAY 360

Write a short letter of gratitude to a teacher or mentor who changed your life. What impact did they have?

"Reality is largely negotiable. If you stress-test the boundaries and experiment with the 'impossibles,' you'll quickly discover that most limitations are a fragile collection of socially reinforced rules you can choose to break at any time."

- Tim Ferriss

DAY 361

What is one thing you can eliminate from your life that would improve it the most?

DAY 362

When you have a great idea, how do you capture it? How can you get better at remembering your ideas?

DAY 363

If you don't believe in yourself, who will? How can you build a fierce self-belief muscle?

DAY 364

Would you rather suffer the pain of discipline or the pain of regret? What does this say about how you should live your life?

DAY 365

What separates men from boys? Is it age, or something more?

DAY 365 AND ¼

What are the 5 most important questions you encountered in this journal? Skim through the questions and pick them out. What do they tell you about who you are as a man, who you could be, and what you really want in life?

"We need the iron qualities that go with true manhood. We need the positive virtues of resolution, of courage, of indomitable will, of power to do without shrinking the rough work that must always be done."

- **Theodore Roosevelt**

Final Note:

Congratulations! You made it. You are now a certified, bonafide, badass man.

How does it feel? Give yourself a moment to celebrate.

When you're done, there's some work waiting for you. Along with your accomplishment comes a call to action.

What will you do to spread the word, and help others on their path towards becoming better men? If you got value here, a review would help this book reach others who can benefit from it.

Because the world needs more men who can face hard times with courage, honor, and kindness.

Made in the USA
Las Vegas, NV
21 December 2022

63624293R00122